I Forgot That You Existed
(Neurological amnesia)

Sophia Le

I Forgot That You Existed

Dedication

To my grandpa, Canh Ha, for being strong even in the toughest and confusing moments.

I Forgot That You Existed

"The burden of a memory is never just filled with despair, it is the emptiness that questions how everything has changed."

Sophia Le

I Forgot That You Existed

I Forgot That You Existed

Table of Contents

Prologue (7)

Chapter 1: Alcohol intoxication (9)

Chapter 2: Wernicke-Korsakoff syndrome (15)

Chapter 3: Working memory (21)

Chapter 4: Retrieval (25)

Chapter 5: Confabulation (29)

Chapter 6: Anterograde (34)

Chapter 7: Strokes (37)

Chapter 8: Death (39)

Epilogue (43)

Author's Note

I Forgot That You Existed

I Forgot That You Existed

I Forgot That You Existed

I Forgot That You Existed

prologue.

Memory loss. Scientifically, it would be called "neurological amnesia". In other words, it's a fancier way to say that you have lost a part of yourself. Your life is forgotten. In this case, this memory loss comes from the damage of the brain activity.

The limbic system. The sphere of influence. Melting into almost nothingness. Shoved and buried. You're alive but not alive. Everything is disoriented. What is even real? *Are these people my family? Where am I? What is happening? Who are you? Who am I?*

White. White. White. White. *White light. Shattering the deepest spikes of your wellbeing. Panic explodes and then all*

I Forgot That You Existed

of a sudden you're the smallest thing in the room. Get. Me.

Out. I can't get out.

"I need you to stay calm." The nurse stares back like it is the most casual thing in the world.

I Forgot That You Existed

1.

Alcohol intoxication. Humans like to feel good. They want to be pleasured and feel warm inside. These hormones bring out positivity. Sometimes, this is present when you are going out with your friends and family or even getting new clothing. What happens when your positivity depends on self harm?

First, it's just for fun. Then you need a couple more. I mean, what's the harm? *Your life.* So then, the question becomes: Is it worth it? *No, of course not.* But you can't stop. The damage has already flowed and

I Forgot That You Existed

consumed. So, might as well keep going then. *It burns. So good.* What happens when your life's on the line?

It's just a drink. You wanted a drink. You *need* a drink. *It's going to be fine.*

Accept it's not. Humans have a hard time rejecting what makes them feel whole and good, even when it is the most harmful thing ever. Deep down, you just want to be seen, to relate to sometime. *To be able to lean back on something.* Logic or not, not everything in this world is a sure thing and nothing is guaranteed. But alcohol never changes, it will always give you the same feeling. So then, what happens when you can't take it much more?

The pain, depression, anxiety and panic attacks. It can be wiped away with a drink. But then it

I Forgot That You Existed

becomes every day. *How much are you willing to lose?* At least with alcohol, the pain is numb. You feel better about yourself, confident even. That's the goal. *To just forget.*

It was only meant to be for a moment. Not a lifetime.

Pain is only momentary. But humans will rarely remember this. We live in the moment, and in the moment where it feels like the world is ending, nothing can be stopped. It becomes out of our control.

The ache takes over, *what is the point of anything?* One thing after another and then your head is pounding.

I Forgot That You Existed

Thump thump thump. *It's in my head.* Unescapable torture surrounded by neverlasting agony. It hurts now, but is it worth the lifetime of never ending torture?

You don't really know until you start to slip away. It then becomes too late.

Thump thump thump. *My heart can't stop beating from this. Panic.* Surely, the drinks would make it go away.

It keeps getting worse. Isn't it supposed to get better?

Can't I stop? Do I even want to stop? How can I stop when this is my only lifeline? Nothing is waiting for me on the other, sober side.

I Forgot That You Existed

It gets better. Except it isn't guaranteed. *Hatred. I'm so sick of myself, I wish I could be anyone else.*

I could be anyone I want to be intoxicated. After all, it is going to help me.

"You're rotting slowly." "You're slipping away from us." "You need to stop." "You need to seek help." "You're choosing the alcohol over your own family." "When is this phase of yours going to end?" "You're going to die."

What's wrong with me rotting?. You were never there to begin with. I can't stop. I know how to help myself. I'm choosing myself. What makes you think this is a phase? Then let me die.

I'm losing them. You've already lost yourself. So why would I try?

I Forgot That You Existed

Then, your head won't stop spinning and making noise. It's moving like a circle. It's a cycle of regret and numbing torment. Over and over again. Spiraling into the unknown, burning the person you are.

Unfortunately, circles are a never ending cycle of agonizing persecution.

I Forgot That You Existed

2.

Wernicke-Korsakoff neurological syndrome. This is caused when there isn't enough vitamin B1 (thiamine).

The Wernicke part refers to the logic of how brain disorders that include alcohol abuse are caused by the decreasing of thiamine. In which, this severely harms the brain's thalamus and hypothalamus.

On the other hand, Korsakoff's syndrome is most closely related to alcoholism. It affects the memory in various ways that damages the brain and the spinal cords and its nerve cells. This includes the part of the brain involved with memory. In this case, the biggest and most important symptom resulting from this comes from amnesia.

There is no treatment for amnesia. Persons under amnesia live a lifestyle in which they have to deal with the fact that they are just simply confused. Oftentimes, this is painful because their mental wellness ceases to exist. It can even lead to physical violence to those around them because they are angry at being in the dark.

The dark after the alcohol. *The dark that they put themselves into.* Who really is to blame then?

Even after the damage is done, the person is still a breathing, living human being. To save all lives is to do everything to help all lives. With no direct or specific research in order to create a life changing cure, all is lost.

Memories make up who a person is. Without it, the person is lost. Their brains keep these forgotten memories behind a lock. The key is thrown into nothingness, and the person is more than likely never going to have access to the key again.

This key holds the power to give someone their potential back. Being kept away behind a barrier from these significant memories eventually becomes a pool of darkness. Whoever is behind the barrier drowns in the end. But if there was a way to bring them back to land, there is a far greater chance that the person is able to emotionally and physically heal. With nothing done, nothing to help, it is forever

I Forgot That You Existed

guaranteed that the person will die, and not as themselves, but as the shell of who they once were.

More trials, more accurate research, more medication, more funds, more being done would be able to save lives.

Isn't it the person's own fault for alcohol binging in the first place? What's more important? The blame or the power to help? Ultimately, it comes down to this: who are doctors choosing to help? What is being prioritized when change needs to be made?

The brain under amnesia is a ticking time bomb. It then goes on to hurt those closely related to it. When it explodes, there is nothing left that can be done. When the brain shuts off into death and darkness, there is nothing left that can be done.

I Forgot That You Existed

Would you want to be a shell of a human in your own body? Would you want to be looked at like a ghost haunting the living?

People under neurological amnesia have no idea what happened, how they got there.

It is a void of darkness waiting to be uncovered.

Second chances are a revival of what could've been. What can be done.

Through grief, acceptance is hard to reach and obtain. Watching life fade away, whether through a first or third perspective is a wash of fear and vulnerability that is inevitable.

There is an answer to every solution, a way to reverse damage.

I Forgot That You Existed

A waiting game is far more dangerous because the outcomes that follow it are indescribable, unethical and unforeseen.

I Forgot That You Existed

3.

Working memory. The spontaneous recall. It leaves faster than it comes. It's almost as if it lightly touches the person before discarding the feeling (or memory) instantly. *Gone and forgotten.*

The working memory retains a new memory for a short amount of time, usually minutes, before the memory vanishes as if it was never there in the beginning.

It's like the trick of the light, a sudden blink, a wave of confucian and mystery.

Though this may seem normal or even useful to the average person, it can be incredibly frustrating to those who have already lost so much of who they are.

He doesn't remember who I was. He thought I was my mother. How could he forget that he had been such a huge part of my childhood? Who I was? Everything he's done for me?

Even still, the echo of his voice calling out my mother's name in my direction still haunts me. It's chilling, to see the ghost of who was once my favorite person. Staring back behind the eyes that shed nothing new is like watching a dying snake shed its skin for the final time.

The wisp of nothingness letches upon his face, as sorrow is reflected off of mine and reflected onto my dreaded mother's face.

I Forgot That You Existed

He was too far gone. Lost in the moonlight even as his breath still lives on.

How this was fair was beyond me.

Even so, I remember not even being able to look at him. It was too terrifying. I was too scared.

"It wasn't him."

I kept telling myself that over and over again. In order for the guilt to be pressed deep down within me.

I needed to justify my grief.

Poor working memory prevents the average person from simply existing in everyday life.

The information comes and goes, a flicker of the light that leaves as fast as it comes.

I Forgot That You Existed

What if the person under amnesia just simply wants to know? To understand. To sympathize. To feel.

The working memory needs to be studied, can it reach its fullest potential?

Can it be tweaked to benefit those who have already lost so much of their own true selves?

I Forgot That You Existed

4.

Retrieval. Sometimes the memory comes back and hits the person like a boulder. Sometimes they feel as if they are the boulder between bliss and the locked, kept memories.

Sometimes the person becomes conscious again of what is going on. Who they are.

Maybe, they're not lost after all. Or maybe, they are just on the edge of remembrance and being disoriented.

Snippets of their own life and the confusion of their state comes. And who knows if it will

I Forgot That You Existed

disappear again. It could be anything or anyone important to them before they had become *lost*.

Or, it was just irrelevant or made no sense to others around them.

It could be almost a flash of fresh air or a glimpse of something that was quickly terminated.

Is it even real? How long had it taken for just one small thing to come back?

It could cost eternity for it all to come back. And no one has eternity to wait.

When does it end? Does it end?

The ringing bell that whispers the name of *death* is unspoken. Though it is unspoken, it is the loudest noise in the room. A mutual understanding as the ghost in laying there continues to decay.

I Forgot That You Existed

The rattles and the chills that echo the unforeseen, yet expected future.

Glances of sorrow become the new mutual form of communication.

He got my mom's name correct this time. It wasn't directed at me any more.

The pang feeling of anxiety floats freely into the sky as the bits and pieces become coherent.

But everyone knows that the surge always happens before the shake of the ultimate breath happens.

No, it must be different in this case.

It's never different.

Are the living souls that surround the corpse just another victim of false hope?

Are they being tricked by the one that is too far gone?

I Forgot That You Existed

The inch of light depicted by the display of small reminisce is no match for the rotten darkness within.

"He must be getting better." They said, and I had no idea if they were trying to convince me or themselves.

I sure didn't believe them.

Maybe, maybe it was manifestation.

The sorrows of "It's going to be okay." That my mother repeats is daunting rather than comforting. And I found that the silence of breath is all I wanted to hear.

The ringing in the room never stopped.

I Forgot That You Existed

5.

Confabulation. When the brain tries to have a filler in memory details but makes a mistake.

It makes a mistake to replace something that was never there.

Again, a ghost of nothingness.

And again, it's not anything new.

An error. A mistake that is impossible to correct.

It's not just a once or twice *issue*. Instead, it is a neurophysic disorder.

The patient doesn't even know they're telling lies.

I Forgot That You Existed

This could range from names of their children and parents to even false made up detailed stories of their life that never even happened.

The holes in the memory are filled with deluded little pieces that just never seem to stop.

At the same time, opposing the patient may result in a crash out.

A breakdown.

Because they too need answers.

They too want to be *fixed*.

The traumatic brain injury, resulting in a wave of something counterfeit.

The false memory is a killer shark.

The undetected deception eats away without the patient realizing.

I Forgot That You Existed

So why does this happen?

Can it be fixed?

Can studies be done to prevent that the brain might not be too far gone?

Or are they just lost causes?

The brain is the most fragile body part in a human's body.

One mistake and the patient's entire life is changed forever.

So it can be seen through the course of history that this fragile part shouldn't be largely invaded.

However, shouldn't there be more done for these patients who live day by day through anxiety and agony?

I Forgot That You Existed

Throughout the course of history, more and more cures, vaccines, medication continue to be developed to treat those who are in need.

Yet anything related to the brain ceases to exist.

Though this is understandable, patients are suffering.

The worst part is that their suffering isn't even physically seen until the *worst* comes.

The mental agony never leaves.

It affects everything within.

It just so happens that the within in question is inescapable with terror.

It's triggering, as the errors are spontaneous.

Expect the unexpected. As they say.

I Forgot That You Existed

Except, just how far can the unexpected go?

In occurrence, the patient can get physically violent. Their thought processes are jumbled and they often don't know what they're doing.

The violence can come in forms of attacks, struggle and even verbally.

Even today, though there is psychological violence that comes from these attacks, it is unknown where this truly reels from.

The mechanism from the brain is unallocated, and thus, is still a mystery today.

6.

Or sometimes. The patient doesn't even know what's going on at all.

Anterograde.

The awakening of the corpse that cannot recall.

Through anterograde, the remembrance does not come from recent knowledge; past memories are more easily able to come by.

The anterograde can be seen as the avoidance of one's current problems.

The beating around the bush, to distract oneself from the ultimate downfall or grievance.

I Forgot That You Existed

This particular type of amnesia is almost like the final ticking of the bomb.

The warning before the end.

Everyone knows this time.

He's already dead.

And again, no one wants to say it out loud.

Instead of moving forward, the person is rooted to one part of their lives.

Repeating over and over again.

The cycle is continuous, asking the same questions again and again.

Until it just stops.

I Forgot That You Existed

7.

Strokes. This can occur when there is a blockage in the brain that is not able to dissolve. In which, the blood is not able to flow to the brain at a normal rate.

The brain can possibly disintegrate and then the rotting decay would start.

This medical emergency can change the life of the patient forever.

Often, this is where it might start. The sorrow is all built up for this dreaded anticipation.

The body becomes weaker and weaker.

I Forgot That You Existed

The state of the body then becomes unpredictable. Anything could happen.

Whatever it is, it then becomes the start of the dominoes that are about to fall.

His body had shook non stop, and the rumble of his bones transferred onto my chattering teeth.

This moment had changed everything.

This was the final switch of the person I used to know. Yet I knew deep down that the signs were present throughout my entire childhood.

The rage.

The break outs.

All of this anger transferred into ultimate demise. My blood ran cold, and the little girl that lived deep inside me

I Forgot That You Existed

sobbed as she had hoped for this wish. She had never dealt with such emotions. This was the start of her pain.

Numbness.

Weakness.

Long term disability is a possible result, in which this is the end of the patient's conscious life and the beginning of an end. *This is more common than brought to light, and it is the center of the loved ones lives.*

I Forgot That You Existed

8.

I remember the exact moment my mom had gotten the call because she had rarely ever shed a tear, much less sob loudly. It was the most chilling sight I had ever seen because I had only seen her cry a total of 4 times in my entire life.

I had school that day. Even so, my mom couldn't help but allow the words to slip from her lips.

It was then that I was sure that my world had crashed.

I didn't speak a word of it to anyone all day. Even as I felt my heart thumping in long overdue denial. There was quite literally no way that this was happening to me.

It was inevitable.

I Forgot That You Existed

So then why did my heart clench around a thousand needles at once when I knew this was coming.

He was already dead before I had even seen him.

I had already lost him as soon as he had hit that hospital bed.

Even still in this moment, I could not get myself to cry.

I had refused to even think about it because I had felt so guilty. There was no recollection of memories, because there were almost none to remember anymore.

The only thing that I could even remember was not saying goodbye. I had never used my last opportunity to even look at him because I was terrified. I was terrified of the corpse that was already dead.

The ghost of my eyes revved to the floor.

The hospital floor.

I Forgot That You Existed

The clinic floor.

The bedroom floor.

My neck couldn't stop bending forward, hunching my back into a corner of bare existence and the exaggeration of my spine burned as my head spun into a million circles.

And if I didn't know better, I would have never registered the chills that the shrunken and shaken body had given me.

Even still, he was alive in my head because my whole house was filled with his life.

The funeral was filled with blurred faces. Those of which I had believed to be frauds.

I Forgot That You Existed

Maybe I should've cried.

Maybe, it would've been easier.

The force of their orbs dilating into waterworks was almost a pathetic sight.

As I kneeled, even then it did not feel real.

My body shook because I wanted it to end.

Yet, I didn't even know how it even ended.

My feet took me to places that I did not recognize, and it wasn't home because it was missing a living soul.

So maybe, it had not been meant to be.

It was a full moon that same night.

Goodbye

Goodbye

Goodbye.

I Forgot That You Existed

epilogue.

I didn't know who I was or what was going on. The sight of the unknown woman in front of me who called herself the nurse simply pissed me off further.

There was an accident.

My skin isn't mine.

My face is blurred.

I couldn't feel my body.

Sleep came, and it never left.

I Forgot That You Existed

I Forgot That You Existed

author's note.

Thank you so much for taking your time to read this book. It means so much to me because it is my own version of a memoir to the bestest friend I've ever had, my grandpa. He, who had gone through all of the stages written in this book, is the strongest fighter I have ever seen. Even in death, he is still my best friend, my drive and love for writing. This (intentionally) short book is not meant to give a professional viewpoint of what patients experience. It is simply my own take and experience. The goal of this book was to relate to others, who have felt the same heartache that I have felt. If there is at least one

I Forgot That You Existed

person reading this book who has reached the end who's heartstrings were struck, then I will know that I have accomplished something with my time.

Thank you Ms Kuga for believing in my skills, potential, and abilities for everything, even when I never believed in myself. Thank you for always sticking by my side and bothering me until I was confident in myself. You are the reason why I'm proud of my writing. You are the reason why I have pushed myself continuously to keep going, even when I was ready to drop everything and crawl into a rotting hole.

I Forgot That You Existed

Thank you Mr Quintero for being the voice of reason, yet never failing to ease the tension or bring a smile to my face. Though your class was extremely easy, you have taught me so much as a person. Thank you for being the teacher I will always have to turn to and seek for help when I'm trapped. Thank you for supporting me through every decision I make, and always showing excitement.

I want to give a special thanks to my best friend, Angelly, who aided me in producing the book cover itself. She has supported me from the very beginning before the book was even written, and when it was all just a jumble of words and my confused brain not knowing where to even start. Oftentimes, the process

I Forgot That You Existed

of writing this short book made me want to quit. Yet, you have never doubted me once. Thank you for being there when I need a shoulder to lean on or just annoy for everything.

I take comfort in thinking that my grandpa, who had endured so much pain, is now able to rest in peace. However, the same cannot be said for patients in the multiple stages (chapter titles) of this book. I hope that this book will be able to change that, that there will be more done to help those who are suffering. The ultimate goal had never been to seek a place to vent. The goal was to ensure that the suffering is cared for.

I Forgot That You Existed

I Forgot That You Existed

www.ingramcontent.com/pod-product-compliance
Lightning Source LLC
Chambersburg PA
CBHW072002210526
45479CB00003B/1033